I0414946

Daniel Staite

EMPATHIC HEALING

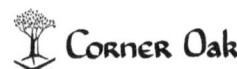

PRESS • PUBLICATIONS • EDITORIAL • REPRESENTATION
Austin and McDade, Texas

© MMXI Daniel Staite. All rights reserved to author.

Published by Corner Oak Press, Publications, Editorial, and Representation,
a branch of The Corner Oak
P.O. Box 143144
Austin, TX 78714
www.corneroak.com

Daniel's Web site is
www.thehealingstate.com

Cover illustration by Zane Staite

First edition
May 2011

Printed in the United States of America

*To my wife Sara
and my children Lauren and Zane.
Thank you for being there with me.*

Foreword

I wrote this book to remind us of our true nature and what we should truly become.

Eugenie and Hannah are two people dear to my heart. They do their best to heal all who are around them.

Unfortunately, they are hurting their own lives in the process. They tend to be adversely emotionally affected after they heal friends.

This is why I have written *Empathic Healing*. Healing should be fun, not detrimental to your life.

Acknowledgments

No one can publish a book like this without the help of friends and colleagues. I'd like to thank my nana, Eugenie Gosselin.

Thanks for the gentle reminders and drive of my Best GFFs, and to Ann Kastetter Davila for copy-editing the rough draft. Finally, thanks to Lindsey Eck of The Corner Oak for final editing, design, and layout.

Contents

Foreword v

Acknowledgments.. vi

Who is Empathic Healing for?... 1

    Maladies.. 4

The Basics 7

The Multi-Layered Bodies 11

    The Chakras.. 14

Keystones.. 19

Protecting the Bodies... 23

    Shielding the Bodies.. 25

    Quick Fix.. 27

Keeping It All Balanced.. 29

    Prayer and Blessings... 30

Cleansing... 33

    Intent and the Heart Chakra...................................... 34

    Fill the Empty Space... 36

Be in the Moment 41

    The Mind.. 42

    Cleansing 49

Salt **50**

Protections **53**

Protection of the Mind, Body, and Creations **53**

Shielding **58**

Psychic Globes **59**

The Aura **60**

Light Shielding **61**

Home and Office **61**

Understanding **63**

The Techniques of Empathic Healing **63**

Let's Get Started Healing **65**

Glossary **85**

Index **89**

About the Author **91**

More from Daniel Staite **92**

Who is Empathic Healing for?

Empathic healing happens naturally in everyday circumstances. We often heal empathically without even realizing it. Some examples:

- Have you ever entered a building and found a rush of energy or pressure upon entering? Did it leave as you left the building? Did it shape your whole day? Did you notice that it even affected others who were not there with you?

- When sitting down to a wonderful dinner in a restaurant, did you experience the painful feeling of a full stomach? Did the guilt of overeating happen even before you started eating? Did it subside and allow you to enjoy the meal, or did it worsen as you ended the meal?

- Healing establishments like hospitals, doctors' offices, and clinics are places with a lot of sickness and anxiety. Has there been a time when you left feeling worse than you did when you arrived? Did that feeling manifest as a physical signal like an itch or a rash?

- Have you gone to a funeral for someone in your interpersonal circle and felt others' grief? Was the grief so real that it clouded your mind? This could be the same as reacting to a violent injury or attack that someone else endures—you have a physical reaction such as grief or anger to the event.

- Have you ever wanted to pay for someone's life choices and thoughts? For instance, at a store you notice that the person ahead of you does not have enough money. Would you pay to alleviate the pain of embarrassment and relieve the pressure in your own body?

- Seeing the struggle of learning something new in some people is a massive problem. It is not always easy to watch people step out of their box. We just need to be patient with them and wait for their minds to catch up with ours. Do you feel their frustration and then become frustrated yourself?

- Have you felt someone else's physical pain, like somehow getting another's headache or backache when you are nearby? Have you felt the pain of a pet, or a wounded wild animal's panic or other emotion? Does the sound of a baby crying give you the baby's unease and confusion or cause you to panic?

- What about happy events like a wedding or visiting an amusement park? Have you felt complete joy the way it actually was, or the opposite of what was expected? Did you feel the excitement of the rides or was fear boiling? Did you feel the pleasure of walking down the aisle and becoming one, or nervousness from something being imperfect?

- Have you gone out to lunch with a friend who had a problem? You sat and listened and, when lunch was over, your friend felt so much better as you walked away with pain in your heart. Without realizing it, you took your friend's emotional pain and issues.

If you answered "yes" to any of these scenarios, then *Empathic Healing* was written for you.

We have all had these experiences. This kind of empathy is not healthy, but it is easy to take on. The problem with healing in this way is that we have no protection. If the pain or issue that we take into our body matches an unlearned lesson within ourselves, then we tend to hide another's problem and make it our own. This energy or emotion will reside in our body, causing us to become sick with our friend's issues and problems over time.

We are all healers, whether we know it or not. Most of us heal others automatically, rather than doing it consciously when we are in the moment and are mentally and emotionally balanced. This is a reminder for you, my family and friends. Empathic healing is for you and perhaps for someone who is dear to you.

We tend to run in a herd and have a close pack of friends. We also have lots of not-so-close people in our lives who move on as quickly as they arrive. You will see that many go as soon as we put them back on their path. We tend to have friends that need our emotional help and support. They unconsciously move forward when they have healed. For our friends to move on is very common when we heal properly. We will see that friends will reenter our life to be healed. We will find that our old friends who assisted us in unlearned lessons will come to us in thoughts, in person, or electronically so that we may heal these wounds. As our patterns change, so too do our thoughts, dreams, and motivations.

Maladies

Have you healed improperly? If so, what has been affected in your life? Are your life, friends, and relationships in a state of awe? Are you fulfilled with work, with your life, and financially? These are things that will improve through the art of self-healing.

When we heal improperly, we can be affected in ways that are hard to understand. I will explain some of the different aspects and feelings that can be by-products of improper techniques so that you can see the broader picture behind the scenes.

We are empathetic beings and this naturally creates a passion for healing. When the healing is felt in unloving or imbalanced ways, healers create problems for themselves. These problems show up in many different ways:

- changing thought patterns
- changes in nighttime dreams and daydreaming
- different people appearing in your thoughts
- worsening of normal body aches and pains
- muscle stiffness
- weight gain
- injuries shortly after experiencing emotions
- emotions running wild, or out of balance
- emotions you have never felt before
- changes in your life's spiritual aspects

We are here to heal ourselves and others. Healing is one of life's greatest gifts, so keep it up. If all humans start healing, the great spiritual awakening will begin. Wouldn't it be just as easy to train us to heal instead of getting angry or upset? Why don't we heal all life lessons we were taught as children? We are able to heal conversations, words, and emotions of the people around us. With empathic healing we will heal others with knowledge that was part of the original design. It takes very little time to improve our lives and the lives of others. The part of the mind we call the unconscious tries to mend itself in many ways. There are clues that show us when we have energetically taken in something that needs to be expelled. For one thing, our dreams start to change visually, in subject matter, or in volume. We have a pattern to our healing. We need to pay attention when this pattern changes. The thoughts that run in the undercurrent of our minds are signs of who we are and what we create in our life experiences.

The issues we are working with are the thoughts we are thinking. So, when your thoughts, dreams, or inspirations alter, then there is a change that needs to be addressed.

If the thoughts you are having are negative, then you are in need of healing, which necessitates lots of self-observation. Our thoughts create our words; thus, words are the tuning forks for the body.

The words we speak create our lives and bodies. Our life experiences are manifestations of how we are known and described. Words are a tool for creation. What you and others say about you creates a vibration that affects you. We are affected by intention, thoughts, and words. In the healing world, these equate to energy, frequency, and vibration. We may change who we are just by acceptance, which changes our life visions. Watch your changing thoughts, actions, and words, for they are your creative power.

Learn to use this power for your own healing as well as for those around you. Watch what you say and keep your words and thoughts positive. This is a great way to start healing your own vibration. When talking to people, keeping your words positive keeps you from being too attached to negative emotions. Positive minds lead to healthier bodies. Do not get caught up in negative emotions; rather, live by actions of peace and compassion. Do not let others feed off your emotions. It is so common that we start out having a wonderful day and others' lives or emotions affect and drain us. By healing others you will still have a great day. The steps of positive thought and healing will lead us to the basics of empathic healing.

The Basics

Empathic healing is a simple technique used to heal those around us. This technique is not new to any of us, and we frequently make use of it without our conscious awareness—and often without proper protection. We are born with natural protection, but most of us disable it in childhood. Establishing protection is a key factor in this healing modality.

I will teach about the original protection for your body and how to restore it. I will cover how to protect the self from other people's unwanted thoughts and energies, which are not healthy for our bodies. Self-protection from all unbalanced energetic items is the foundation of this chapter; their proper handling and disposal are also important.

Empathic healing is very simple and easy to learn. Those who have learned to do it properly do so with very little thought. The rewards you receive from healing are priceless. The joy you receive will last a lifetime. I've come to find that most people are carrying others' emotions. That isn't necessarily bad, but most of those emotions are negative. This burden bearing is causing a lot of unnatural health problems. People do not need other people's sickness. Yet we see family members passing the flu or a cold back and forth. We have seen one person's stress transferred throughout a whole office. Stress is known to be part of most people's illness. Stress weakens the aura and natural defenses against infection and viruses. A major constraint is that we were taught how to react to stressors improperly, resulting in an imbalance in our etheric fields that can be reduced or removed easily through empathic healing.

I am writing to teach how to heal empathically without becoming ill from other people's problems. All who use this technique will be able to heal their friends and families. While healing others, you automatically start healing yourself. When the people you rely on most are healthy, you naturally become healthier and stronger with less negativity in your body.

Life will start to become very easy. All that is needed to be a healer is a little love and faith. I hope this intrigues your mind and your heart.

Empathic healing will open your heart, challenge your mind, and purify your spirit. If you have been looking for a quick and easy healing technique, you have found it. Empathic healing is based on love. Love has started wars and it has ended them. We have all experienced having a friend cry on our shoulder as we sat and listened. Our spending time with such a friend is healing and soothing in itself. I know a way that we can heal empathically, and no one will know that it is occurring. Handshakes or hugs are as much touching as you will need to give. You will learn how to use your heart and intention to heal those who are around you. All you will need is a little time to practice. With friends and family like mine, you will find a lot of people coming to you for help. What do we need to cover before we start healing?

- An explanation of the physical and energetic bodies
- Basic knowledge of the chakras and how they work
- The link between auras and chakras and how they work

There are many ideas and philosophies about the energetic aspect of humans. I need only cover the basics for you to be able to heal properly. What is most important is that you are able to heal without taking in that which you are removing from others. I hope and believe that all will want to make this healing technique a part of their daily lives, healing all with whom they come into contact. That will change the greater vibration and consciousness of humanity and all that is around us.

The gift of healing is a treasure far greater than monetary abundance. It is the easiest step on the path to enlightenment of one's body, mind, soul and sprit. This healing path will bring great karmic wealth as well as personal abundance and stature. You will start to think differently and seeing the world around you in a different way. The morning will start easier with less hassle to get out the door. Work will be a place of enjoyment for you and those you work with daily. The family home will be a place of laughter and harmony. Relationships will become easy. Ways to create or make extra money will come in a constant and easily flowing manner. Healing others is enjoyable in so many ways. I know you will gain as much pleasure from this path as I have.

The Multi-Layered Bodies

The physical human body is composed of many organs and systems that have elements of layering. Examples include the epidermis, tendons, ligaments, and the muscular, nervous, and circulatory systems. The energetic body is interlaid into the physical body and is also a multi-layered system. I will give a quick overlay of the human body as we know it physically and energetically, briefly explaining some of the functions and properties of these bodies.

You don't need to be knowledgeable about the body and each of its functions to perform this mode of healing. We only need to understand that there is a life lesson that is imbalanced. The body itself does its own healing naturally. There are times when slight guidance will make an enormous difference. I will assist you in understanding that the purpose of healing is to remove lessons and to allow another's body to heal.

If you step on a piece of glass, you can remove the glass and the body will heal naturally. The same is true for all emotional lessons. If you leave the glass in, the body will heal around it but unnecessary pain and impurity will remain.

The physical body is what we see, feel, and know. The thought of who I am is more than physical—it is spiritual. When we define ourselves as the body, we know that our words and thoughts are what create the life we live. The words we speak are vibrations. Thoughts are electrical impulses in the brain. We are now leaving the physical and moving into the etheric aspects of the body. That is why the next section is important. Understanding that there is a lot more to us than the body should help us separate from the emotional aspect of this world, which in turn will assist us in our ability to heal so that the client or friend who is being healed does not affect us. Here is how the bodies start to change from physical to the etheric.

The liquid body carries nutrition to the other bodies. The liquid body is in tandem with the plasmic body; as one flows, so does the other. The liquid body carries the nourishment to the physical body's cells. The plasmic body carries the energy to the etheric side of the bodies. It also carries gaseous material through the physical body. The liquid body is layered tightly with the gaseous body. The gaseous body helps nourish the etheric, liquid, and physical bodies. The connection between the gaseous, liquid, and etheric bodies is where the plasma material resides. The etheric body nourishes all the bodies with *chi*, or *prana*: energy that resides in all aspects of life. The etheric body pushes and pulls this energy through doors or wheels known as *chakras*. I see these doors as energy bubbles.

The superetheric body is where the spirit and soul are connected to all aspects of the other bodies. Here is where energy and vibration begin to form conscious matter. This is the body where memories are stored in amino acids. The subatomic body is where energy flows through the body in a layer under the physical structure.

This body works with cells' growth, programming, and movement. It controls the plasma material that manifests into the visible identifiers of the physical body. The atomic body is where consciousness and thought reside, and where thought waves are converted into brain functions. It is where mind—superego, ego, and id—becomes an aspect of higher identification.

This empathic healing technique uses the etheric body to pull and remove energies from people to start their healing process. This technique is very minute and is invisible to the naked eye for most people. Still, you may be able to tell when someone is working on you or when others are being worked on. It can be detected by the physical movement of one's body in response to the pulling of energies. Patients may tend to rock forward and backward when you work on them. Sometimes there are dramatic emotional changes in the person who is being worked on. Most people do not observe their bodies or emotions closely enough to notice these types of changes. For you as a healer, these changes will start to become part of your understanding of the healing process—and besides, they serve to validate the great healing that you are doing.

Empathic healing uses love to heal all those who are around us. We use the etheric body to pull chi or prana through the chakras and release emotions and negative thoughts. I like to call negative thoughts facets of life's unlearned lessons. We will pull unlearned lessons from people and assist in their healing.

The Chakras

Chakra is defined as 'wheel'. All of the renderings I have seen of chakras are of a flattened top view. Distinct elements, sounds, frequencies, emotions, bodies, petals, stars and colors are associated with each of the major chakras.

A major chakra measures about 6 inches or larger, minor chakras 3 to 5 inches. Miniscule chakras measure 2 inches or less. Most books state there are seven major chakras, but there are actually more. Any person who is slightly athletic tends to have foot, knee, and hand chakras that span more than 6 inches in diameter. There are at least two minor chakras for each major chakra root. The chakras look like floating soap bubbles, with a small vortex that connects the bubbles to the chakra root. A vortex is a whitish swirl, resembling a tornado, that will change direction of spin many times a second. Chakras change colors as they spin. Each chakra has a dominant color. When they are healthy, they can have a beautiful rainbow effect. When they are cluttered with emotional baggage and unlearned lessons, they spin slower and become less brilliant and appear gray.

Chakras work like energetic lungs. They pull in healthy prana (energy) and expel old or sluggish prana. The chakras are attached in pairs to a single root. Major and minor chakras' roots are an organ or bone joint. Chakras spin in opposite directions. The etheric energy inside the organ or joint spins back and forth. The spin makes the energy at the root of the chakra twist and turn. The chakra can now spin fast or slow, depending upon how clean it is. The healthier the chakra, the faster it will spin. The movement of the chakra can release prana or pull it in.

Chi (or prana) energizes the bodies. Chi enters the chakra and spirals into its root, empowering it and energizing the bodies by filling them with aspects of chi. The empowerment also creates an energy field around the bodies as a whole. This field is strengthened by the minor and miniscule chakras. They also support the major chakra and the etheric body. The minor and miniscule chakras make their own fields inside of the fields of the major chakras.

Energy fields will protect. The empowered root creates an energy field or healing partition that is a natural protector from unbalanced energies.

This energy field is commonly called the *aura*, and is also known as an esoteric field. It is a multi-layered field that begins about $1/16$ inch from the epidermis. The chakra roots project each field a little farther away from the physical body the higher from the earth the chakra root is.

The soles-of-the-feet chakras' roots project about $1/16$ inch from the physical body. Each knee chakra's root aura is 2–3 inches from the body, while the energy-field root for the basic and sacral chakras is 9–12 inches away. It is easiest to see the energy fields closest to the physical body. The farther the aura is from the physical body, the harder it is to see—we need a clairvoyant eye. (The clairvoyant eye is the ability to see subtle energy.)

The outer auras have been used by healers for years and are

familiarly called esoteric fields. (*Esoteric* means 'understood by few'.) The esoteric fields are just like their visible counterparts. There are many healing modalities that work with the esoteric fields. In the healing community, most believe that the outer auras begin only 3–4 feet from the physical body, meaning the esoteric fields extend thereafter. In truth, these fields are still part of the aura. They stretch farther than an arm's length and—depending on the energy of the person—possibly miles.

Aura fields have linked chakras. There are chakras in the fields that have counterparts in the bodies. These chakras are connected to the counterpart roots inside of the physical body.

Each level of auras sends energy to all of the bodies. The aura also catches vibrations and frequencies from the bodies. Aura fields have cilia- or hair-like energy that comes off them. This energy is referred to as *health rays*. The rays, like cilia, move unwanted particles off the aura. If the particles do not move, then the health-ray energy starts to break them into even smaller particles.

The health rays receive vibration, energy, and frequencies and integrate them into the chakras. The point where each health ray connects to the aura has a programming marker or emotional aspect. The health rays stick almost straight out from the aura. They slightly sway with the direction in which the chakra root is turning. They will sway back and forth as the chakra root turns back and forth. I have described them as Cousin It (the Addams Family character) with static in his hair or, for the younger crowd, Mike from the *Barnyard* animation. I hope those descriptions help you get a mental picture. Cilia, like health rays, contain plasma material that helps keep them conductive to energies. The plasma also carries the emotions of our body. It attracts like concepts into our life—one of the steps in the law of attraction.

The plasma can escape the health rays under conditions of extreme negative emotions, causing the rays to get stuck, and the aura's body to cease operating properly. When the health rays are damaged they lie down close to the body. When the health rays are lying down, they are not working. Then unwanted energies, particles, or vibrations can enter the aura fields, changing them and their operation. What affects the fields also affects the body.

The vibrations, energies, and emotions that collide with the aura fields affect the conscious mind. We have all entered a room and been able to feel an emotion. The vibration of the emotion affects the plasma in the health rays and signals the bodies. This reaction triggers a response in the physical body because of the learned lessons of our lives. We react to the triggers in the manner that we learned from our lessons. The lessons can trigger an emotional or physical response in either a positive or an unbalanced way.

Strengthening the energetic body supports the physical body. The energetic body creates complex filters and safeguards for our health and emotions. Strengthening the energetic body supplies more prana to all of the other bodies. More prana will strengthen the aura and the emotions protecting us, also creating more emotional balance. It is easier to create manifestations in our lives from a state of emotional balance, or when we live with joy.

Balancing is an act used to repair the aura's fields. It is begun by filling the auras with energy, strengthening them along with the health rays. There are many different types of energy. Most people use white light as the visualization tool to send divine energy. So fill the aura and health rays with white light. Next, pulse the chakras with golden energy to repair damage to the auras and health rays. The golden energy will balance the programming markers, or emotional aspects in the aura and energetic body. The golden energy should come from the crown chakra located above the client's head. Try to use the client's own energy to heal his or her body. The crown chakra is above the physical body and is not easily drained, even when the client is low on energy. The balancing of the aura and the connected fields will assist in easier healing, cleaning, and protection of your bodies as well as those of whoever you are working with. This is an essential part to your own self-healing and protection. When doing this technique to yourself, use the golden energy from the crown chakra above your head.

We are here to make it through life with greater ease and with a grace of being. By doing this simple technique every day you will be able to handle this world's events more calmly and with greater grace.

Keystones

A keystone is a fundamental or basic element of life. It is a stone block that keeps outer stones from falling, usually in an archway.

Keystones in healing are events, actions, or lessons that were not learned correctly. Once a keystone is identified and removed, the other lessons can be removed with ease.

A keystone may be an unbalanced lesson. If you hid under the bed when your parents were angry as a child, you could associate hiding with anger as an adult. Hiding from anger is not acceptable in the work force. One small event experienced earlier in life can change the way one reacts to so many other events in adulthood. One misunderstood statement can create life-changing insecurities such as fear, resentment, lying, shyness, or lack of willpower.

Keystones have changed the bearer's life. The vibration of a keystone will attract the same lesson over and over until it is learned. The lesson in life could have been learned easily had a vibration-attracted balance. Keystones attract life's imbalances. Keystones create a vibration to attract or push away things. If you want abundance and success but are not able to accept them, your inability is due to a keystone pushing the things you want away.

Money does not grow on trees, but if you are an orange farmer it does. Abundance will be found in all things, you just need the wisdom to see how to make it benefit you. Removing a keystone stops the repelling energy so you are able to move forward easily with your plans. Removal of a keystone releases a lot of the stuck, repetitive lessons in that keystone's emotional line of healing and removes or softens the vibration attracting the imbalances in people's lives.

A keystone will change appearances in the mind's eye. I have seen them look like bricks. At other times, they've looked like spheres spinning around each other. This has to do with what role they are playing.

Keystones will block emotions and energy, and may also amplify the emotions so they are running at a high volume. Keystones may be a block to knowledge and wisdom. They might be a spiritual, emotional, energetic, or physical blockage. The difference in their nature tends to leave different appearances in the mind's eye. These appearances are a way to recognize their differences and the techniques needed to heal them.

A keystone may be fulfilled in different ways. Once a keystone and stagnant energy are removed, the resulting open area then needs to be filled. This also may be done in different ways.

The old way involves using colors of light to fill the vacant area. Success would depend on the healer being guided by inner thoughts. Most healers these days are not connected to their inner voice.

We know that white light contains aspects of all colors. I recommend using white to fill the voids. It fills faster and easier when using intention. You do not have to use the inner voice when using this version of the technique.

Another method is to ask clients' spirit and soul to fill the area with their essence—a technique I have devised. I think it is the best method. The request does not have to be out loud, though I do know that spoken words have more power than ones said in your head. I will leave that choice up to you.

Over the past few years I have had great advances in healing using this new version. When I ask I will see the area fill with a brilliant white. I understand most do not see as I do. Have patience and you will feel the energy change in the person you are working on. The energy can get so strong it feels like it is pushing against you.

Invoking divine healing through prayer is a great way to ensure that the area is filled divinely. Just remember: When asking a divine question, wait and feel the reply before moving on to the next step. All prayers are answered energetically before becoming physical. The removal of keystones is a very important aspect of healing. If we neglect their removal and cleansing, then filling, the problems will come back and those being healed will remain stuck. When the keystones are removed, they will be able to let go of unbalanced thought patterns and move forward. A really old pattern might take a couple of healing sessions to be removed, but each session will get lighter and easier.

Stay diligent with the healing and enjoy the process. It is fun to see people blossom in their lives. I am still at awe in all the epiphanies of people who are in my interpersonal circle. I also honor people whom I quietly healed for the great changes in their lives. Once the changes begin, then the process seems to help the healing proceed faster and more easily. Honor yourself for all the changes in their lives. Self-validation is an important tool for healing others. I especially enjoy the work I do when others think they initiated it.

Without the keystone removal, healing will only be emotional and will only last as long as the person's thought patterns are on a different track. Let us heal in the best way we can by keeping ourselves healthy and our interpersonal relationships on a path that is most beneficial for them.

These are simple techniques for a complex cluster of emotions and thought patterns. Practice them and have fun with the healing experience. This is a wonderful and wealthy way of life.

Protecting the Bodies

It is important to understand that all of the bodies need to be protected when healing others. Healers should perform quick maintenance before and after sessions, keeping the balance and strength of all bodies a priority. Meditation and the full healing protocol should be done by themselves weekly. I recommend seeing another healer at least once a month. That also has to do with how much healing you are doing. The more energetically clean you are, the stronger the healing you will be performing, making the healing experience more honoring and rewarding.

To protect the physical body, we need to fill the chakras with golden prana. Each chakra contains aspects of gold. The crown chakra has gold that is plasma. It is thick and coats the aura and health rays, allowing more time for healing. Psychic energy balls or shields are great secondary protections.

The liquid body is protected by the aura fields being covered with plasma gold. Another option is to fill the liquid body with bright white light. This will keep vibrations and frequencies from residing in and affecting the liquid body. A third technique is to keep the liquid body moving. This can be achieved with intent or by being physically active when healing. I understand that is not always possible, so try to imagine 10 jumping jacks if you feel too much energy.

The gaseous body is only affected by emotional vibrations and frequencies. This body stays clean as long as it is not affected for the long term. Protection for the gaseous body is achieved in the same way as for the physical body: by sending gold prana into the chakras. It is a great idea to use this technique right before you start healing someone.

The etheric body is protected when all of the chakras are filled with the crown chakra's plasma gold. It is also protected by static electricity flowing through it. You create this static energy when you are active, or through intent.

The superetheric body is protected by a flow of cosmic energy. This is the divine white light that enters the crown chakra. This body needs to be filled with divine light. It has its own consciousness and is able to balance itself when asked.

Our subatomic body cannot be affected by the healing energies unless the outer bodies are not protected properly. Unbalanced energies have to be integrated into the bodies for the subatomic body to be affected. The integration of these unbalanced energies takes about 72 hours. You will notice the change coming over you, and will be able to recognize that you need to remove the imbalances before full integration is complete.

The atomic body is affected only by thought frequencies and vibrations. This body is protected by keeping your mind and thoughts pure. The best technique for doing so is to fill your thoughts and the person being healed with love. This technique starts the process of empathic healing.

All of these protection techniques for the bodies are natural, innate defenses. I will discuss additional techniques to help create further protection. I recommend doing these techniques as often as possible. Try to use them especially before and after healings. I use the techniques as part of my weekly cleaning protocol. As we are human, we might have blockages in our own bodies or holes in our auras. Holes can be caused by smoke, chemicals, drugs, alcohol, and certain meats. Your body is a wonderful tool and a perfect house. Please honor it by doing that which honors you to the full extent that you are able. Blockages and holes can also be caused by lessons that are learned improperly. I believe that protection is a negative word; I used it only to give examples. As you heal, the protections will become techniques of self-healing, things you do because it feels good to do so. These techniques are here to assist you in becoming healthier and happier in your life.

Shielding the Bodies

You can shield your bodies by creating an energy ball and placing all of your bodies inside of it. I have found that a two-layered ball of pink with gold will block or catch all that you will allow it to. There are issues people share that a healer can accidentally take on if not paying proper attention.

Pull a pink energy ball from your heart chakra, about 8 inches in diameter. Next, pull a 7-inch gold energy ball from your solar-plexus chakra. Place the gold ball inside of the pink one, and then place all of your bodies and minds inside of this ball. I believe in power or key words, using all that I am as I place the ball with myself into the chakra root called *dan tien*. This chakra root sits just below the navel and inside the body. Dan tien is where the body's energy is stored. Integrate the energy ball with the chakra. The energy will feed the shields. You will feel a change of energy throughout your body; wait for it to make sure you have done the technique properly. If you are unsure, ask someone to watch you and see if the body sways slightly.

Empathic healing uses the heart chakra and pulls unbalanced energy into it, so I protect it with a shield. This shield is created from the crown and root chakras. The crown chakra holds the keys to divine and physical elements. Pull a divine energy ball from the crown and let it descend from the top of your head. Feel the divine ball travel down the front of your body into your front heart chakra. The divine ball is an electric, very bright white. Next, take an energy ball from the physical root chakra. This is an esoteric chakra below the feet that is always rooted in the earth. Feel the ball ascend the front of the legs, into the hips, up your back, and through the rear chakras to the heart-chakra root. This sometimes has a warming effect through the whole body.

This energy ball is bronze and changes to gold when it leaves dan tien and ascends to the heart-chakra root. Integrate the two energy balls in the heart-chakra root. Feel the energy change as the balls integrate. Sometimes there can be emotional pain in the heart area as this shield cleans and protects. This is due to its process of cleaning that chakra, allowing those keystones to be removed. I believe that *shields* is a negative-based word. I have used it to give examples. As you heal, the protections will become self-healing techniques, things you do because it feels good. These techniques are here to assist you in becoming healthier and happier in your life.

Quick Fix

I have found an over-the-counter homeopathic product that strengthens the human aura. It is a salt tablet called Bioplasma made by Hyland's. It will boost your aura and your fields. This product will also strengthen the health rays. A dose works for about an hour and a half, though it will wear off sooner if you eat or drink while under its protection. I hope you will find it as effective as I do. As I said, it is a quick fix; using self-healing techniques is a better way to go.

Keeping It All Balanced

When you are balanced, you are less likely to be affected by others' unbalanced energies or vibrations. The best way to maintain this state is to balance the minds, both conscious and unconscious. The doors to these reside in the heart chakra. Send pink or green light from the heart chakra. This will still your presence and enable you to be in the moment, allowing more efficient healing. The combination of pink and green light will soothe and heal at the same time. Try sending the light to yourself and absorb it into your aura for a great calming sensation.

There are times when a friend's lessons are so thick that even more assistance is needed. In this case, create a bonfire with intent. Its size should correlate with the level of demand from the lessons. Imagine a gold and green fire. I normally see it as a gold fire with green tips on the flames. If your inner eye sees changes, let them be. I believe in your inner divinity. While healing, keep your attention on the fire, or it will get smaller, and cut the energy to the fire when you are completed. I have found, when cutting things like fire or energy cords, I can use an implement, which makes the effect stronger mentally and unconsciously. I believe in you and in your healing abilities.

There will be times and places where you need to emotionally shield yourself and others. The color of the fire will combine bronze from the earth chakra and brilliant white from the crown chakra. The flames are bronze and the flickers are brilliant white. Make a circle of fire around the group, or place the group inside the flame to help emotionally clean the group by earth grounding. This technique is great when there are too many emotions and people need to be given a diving force. I have used this in work and group situations when trying to complete a task.

Prayer and Blessings

I am religious and very spiritual. That is my passion. I know all have their own roads, and I love all to believe what they want. Personally, I pray as I start to heal. The prayer ends when I have balanced myself, which is after the session is over. I always ask for blessings, as they are timeless. Blessings are a simple way to teach in an energetic healing session. All people can ask for blessings, and they are always given. The process is very beautiful for a clairvoyant to watch. A brilliant light fills whatever is blessed. Outside of the light a myriad of colors are sparkling. There are energy threads sparking in the object being blessed. It is a sight to behold.

I always ask to have that which was not done correctly be divinely corrected, and to let the person free all that will be most beneficial in life and the healing session. Those who come usually want to be healed for one issue. That may or may not be what is most beneficial for them. I will pull the keystone for this issue because it is my intention to heal all. I heal with the concept that I want these people to become perfect in their own eyes.

We have our own perceptions of what is great and what fulfills us. This is the part of life that is balanced. We all choose different paths due to how such choices make us feel. If we were taught life is easy and abundant, it will be. Most of us were taught that work was something we were not supposed to like, so it is thus. I will say these words a lot: *Do things you like and start to say things you love.*

Pray for a beautiful life with whom and what you want in it. Wait after each prayer and feel the blessing, and be prepared to accept it into your energy. Our prayer amplifies our word, so speak loudly and clearly.

Keep the prayer positive. Be sure of what you want and be prepared to accept the blessing. Try not to be too specific, and enjoy all the things you receive. The gifts you give will go to those who accept more graciously than others. That is just a part of the laws of attraction. Pray often.

Cleansing

I teach meditational breathing, or using controlled breaths. Breathing with intent will help your consciousnesses grasp how this technique works. When you breathe out, you want the front chakras to expel waste and the rear chakras to pull in prana. When you inhale, know that the front chakras pull in prana and the rear chakras are expelling waste. This helps you prepare for healing others. This should be done as part of your weekly maintenance.

Controlled breathing is cleansing for you and your bodies. I recommend a count of 10 or more for breathing techniques. A 10-count technique comprises a four-count inhale, a one-count pause, a four-count exhale, and a one-count pause. Repeat.

When you practice the breathing, feel the bodies pull and push the energy in and out of your chakras. This feeling ensures a more thorough release of waste. When you are releasing waste, memories or thoughts will sometimes get in the way. These memories are lessons that are not understood, or are twisted. Allow them to be freed from your bodies. They are no longer needed. Such a release is an easy way to self-heal the bodies and energies. Sometimes we feel a loss of connection to this energy and these memories. Remember: To free yourself from these imbalances leads to a happier and wealthy life. The more of this energy you clear from your fields and body, the better your health and the clearer your thinking. Remind yourself of this when you feel stuck; it is better to free than to keep yourself contaminated. After all types of sessions, have your spirit and soul fill the vacant area. Please remember: It is easy to keep the old energy; it is awe inspiring without it.

Intent and the Heart Chakra

The heart chakra is the key to empathic healing. When shielded properly, the heart chakra will pull the issue from the friend or patient.

Helping release the issues will help emotions, but that is just a quick fix. It does not heal like removing the original imbalance—the keystone. Removing the keystone will start an avalanche of old imbalances being released. The healer will place the intent or simply think about the energy flow while breathing. Feeling the push and pull of energy in and out of the heart chakra will begin the healing. Allow your mind to enter the process, visualizing all that comes to you. If you are healing someone who knows you are doing this work, tell that person what you see. The visualization and validation become stronger and allow you to become more clairvoyant. Have fun with it—it will validate you the more you are able to do it. There are those people who will deny send them pink and gold from the heart chakra. In time with more healing they will start to change.

I have found that visual markers help in training oneself to be more effective in this process. Here are a few of the ones I use for teaching empathic healing:

1. See the issue as a cloud, smoke, or an object.

2. When released, visualize the issue, or imagine it changing color.

3. See the keystone issue as holding other issues up as in an arch's capstone.

4. Keystones come out with a slight tug; notice their body moving or relaxing.

5. The keystone will change color once it is removed if the removal does not render it golden.

6. See clouds, smoke, or objects follow the keystone in a rock slide.

7. The rock slide should also change color as it is released.

8. Watching golden rocks fall out is excellent.

9. See the golden bricks change into brilliant energy.

When the keystone has turned into brilliant energy, the most important work is completed. I try to see all the energy as a brilliant light when healing others. It makes for a greater healing session. Pull the keystone and see it all turn brilliant white.

I use these visualizations to help healing go deeper and be more complete. Images of energy and emotions help the third eye begin to work more easily. The third eye is the door to clairvoyance—a gift that we all have, but stop using as we grow up due to lessons that we learned improperly. With empathic healing you will start to see the world differently and will also start to see it with clairvoyant eyes.

This is the next level of understanding. Know that clear senses will start to form within you: clairvoyance, clairaudience, and so forth.

Fill the Empty Space

The empty space where the keystones no longer exist needs to be fulfilled. This can be done in a lot of different ways. Here are a couple of techniques. Try them all and see which technique feels the best to you. We all have one that seems to go directly with our personality—have fun with yours.

- *Prayer*

Pray that the area be fulfilled with divine essence and light. Ask that the area always stay pure and filled with light. Ask that all blockages be divinely removed and refilled with light for all time, and that the healing persists divinely. Remember to wait for the prayer to be answered—there will be an energy change in you and the person being healed. This is your choice and your prayer. Use words that feel comfortable to you. My words are not the only ones.

- *Brilliant white light*

This is another great technique to fulfill the open area. Use the light that enters the crown chakra and direct it into the recently vacated area. This helps with the patient's emotional balance —and yours. Allow the area to be fulfilled as much as it takes to glow in your mind's eye. That could take up to 20 seconds—not any more.

• *Golden plasma*

Use the liquid golden plasma from the crown chakra to fill the void left by the removal of the keystones. This will take a lot more mental awareness. The plasma moves slower than light, so it also takes more time to fill the void. This technique is better for people who are depleted of energy. Besides using it for self-healing, you should use it only on people who give their energy to others—those who try to give energetic support to many people.

• *Spirit and soul*

This is my favorite way to fulfill the recently vacated areas. Let their soul and spirit fill the space with their essence and keep it balanced, clean, and divine always.

I have had a lot of great healing sessions with this technique. The honor that you bestow will be returned to you. This may seem a little self-serving, but it feels good when you learn to accept it. I ask the soul and spirit to fulfill where the keystone had resided. The request does not have to be out loud, but is stronger if made orally. I will speak it softly with conviction when working on someone who does not know I am healing him or her. This is a technique that has been taught to me spiritually and has met with wonderful success in my healings.

If we do not fulfill the vacated area, the clients or friends are more likely to pull some of the energy back into their body. Their unconscious minds are trained to follow old patterns. After such healings, I do my best to change these patterns by fulfilling the area. I strongly recommend this conscious pattern in your healing.

Use one technique, or many at the same time. I have said that I pray throughout the healing process. I fill the void with golden plasma as I ask the spirit and soul to fulfill the void as well. That is using three techniques at once. Each session varies, so keep the basic steps, but they do not need to be rules. Taking control is the change you are making in your life. Please take it slow, allowing the techniques to become part of your routine. When you are learning, if you go slow, the steps become easier and help you become stronger in your ability, making healing a pleasure—not a job or a task. The reward will fulfill your life. Practice the self-healing (protections and shields); remove the keystone and see it turn to brilliant light. Fulfill the area that the keystone has vacated. See the light in the mind's eye.

Watch for the body to react subtly to your technique. Validation is performed by being watchful. See the body of the person you are healing move. Feel the energy flow through your body. Sense the changes of energy in the room. See how other people react to the healing even when not consciously knowing. Enjoy the sensation after the healing session. Watch the facial expression of the friend you heal change as you are healing. Emotional outbursts can and will happen. Send your friend the green and pink light from the heart chakra—it will subside in a few moments. By being watch-ful, you will validate your own ability and thus you will not need another to speak for you. This will create a strong confidence in your own healing ability. In no time all will know that you have been right there healing them.

Be in the Moment

To be in the moment is to shut off the clouded thoughts that circle in your mind. This is a technique of clearing the jungle of your life and allowing you to be calm. Fill your heart chakra with pink light. This light will give strength, calm, and balance. Pink light is love and helps you to release life so that you can be in the moment. Being in the moment will help you to hear and see the changes of the patient you are working on. The moment will allow you to adjust quickly to what the other person needs. This begins to allow your intention to assist in a process that would otherwise be totally mental. Free your thoughts, and let the voice from your heart speak to you. Allow yourself to focus only on the voice that resonates in the chest area.

Freeing your thoughts is as easy as healing them. Heal the thoughts with white light and by seeing them turn into energy or disappear. It will take time to free the multiple levels of thoughts that exist in the minds. This is the way to keep you getting closer to being in the moment all the time. There is another method where you see, touch, feel, taste, hear, and smell all the things that are around you. The idea is to keep all things in your senses so you are aware of them, with your minds expanding. During this expansion, the thoughts will quiet and you will start to feel the joy and love of being in the moment. Both of these techniques will assist you in the path of healing and joy.

Being in the moment should be part of our lives. We tend to be so busy in our minds, running errands and making shopping lists, that we stop seeing the world around us. The flowers, the children playing, smiles and laughter of others go blankly unnoticed due to the turmoil in our minds. The moments that stay with us are those where we stopped being in our little world and sat down to be with others. We have lost touch with our friends and family members to create a shopping list that is already written on the counter. When will the world stop focusing on drama to be in the moment? When we start doing so, then joy will become the foundation of our lives.

The Mind

The words we speak create our life and body. Thoughts are the foundation for creation. We are affected by intention, thoughts, and words. In the healing world, these equate to energy, frequency, and vibration. Your thoughts are your intention, the base of your creative power. How have you being laying the foundation of your creativity?

I teach clear senses: using clairvoyance and more. In these classes, I help you understand that when working on clairaudience, you have only one voice. This voice comes from your vocal cords. Your soul's voice radiates from the heart. The voice of your spirit flows from the belly area. So who are these other voices you hear in your head? These are the thoughts of others—or of guides and entities—that you have accepted.

Thoughts are your intention. If the thoughts in your head are not yours, who is creating for you?

Is it time to free some voices?

Prayer

The divine healer is always there to assist you. I have never found the right words to clear more than 10 to 15 percent of the noise at a time. That is still a good amount, and it will take some time to keep the voices to a minimum. When praying, please have the keystone that attaches to the voices removed and fulfilled—to clear the mind, and so that the unconscious will not bring the voices back. The unconscious will otherwise bring the energy and the keystone back because it is programmed to have that noise and energy. We need to reprogram the higher aspects of the mind. It is time to clean them up. We are now beginning the cleanup phase of our life so that our healing ability becomes stronger. When praying, please remember to wait for the answer—whether the person praying can feel the tingle of energy, the warmth of energy, the coolness of a blessing, or pressure around the skin or the aura swelling. All of these are signs that the prayer is being worked on. Always wait to enjoy the answer of divinity.

Meditation

Meditation is another great way to keep the voices down. There are a lot of guided meditations that will assist you in self-healing. There are some that are specially designed to help with your psychological journey. Key words to look for are "quieting the mind."

I have created two CDs (as the beginning of a series) to help anyone learn basic techniques of meditation and visualization, both available from the Blue Oak Record Group:

Meditation for Healing (DS 0901)

Meditation for Interpersonal Relations (DS 0902)

Look for these at <www.cdbaby.com/danielstaite> or at the iTunes store.

I can also recommend:

Meditation on Twin Hearts for Psychological Health and Well Being

There are many more styles and authors. I know with time you will find one that flows with your mind and lifestyle.

Mind healing

This is the meditation technique that I use all the time. I sit and get my body still and relaxed. Then I fill my minds that reside in my chest cavity with the golden liquid plasma from the crown chakra.

The minds in your chest are the conscious ego, the super-conscious soul (or superego), and the unconscious.

I let the golden plasma fill the chest, flow up through the neck into the brain cavity, and then fill the eyes and ears. I let the plasma come out the top of the head so that it starts to cover the body, and then I flood all thoughts with a brilliant white light. I say "heal" out loud three to five times. Then I remove the keystone, have it turn to brilliant light, and fulfill the vacant area.

As I stated earlier, another method is using your senses on things that are around you. Be aware of all things and the minds will start expanding. During this expansion, the thoughts will quiet and you will start quieting the mind. Please use your favorite technique. Remember to use your soul and let your spirit fill the vacant area. Thank you.

I repeat many times until the mind and brain cavity are quiet.

On the go

On the go, I use the same technique, but simplified. When any thoughts enter my head that are not deemed divine, I say "heal" five times and flash the word with a brilliant bright light to quickly heal. I do not always say it out loud. I then remove the keystone with a good exhale, see it turn to light, and fulfill the area with my soul's and spirit's assistance.

I repeat as needed.

You will find, as you move forward in the process of quieting your minds, that others' voices or your interpretations of their thoughts will enter your brain. These will need to be healed as well. Such healing will become protocol after a while. You will find yourself healing others' words as they speak them out loud, which will stop your letting other people's words and powers alter your creation. This kind of healing is one of the best tools to pass on when it comes to creating wealth and abundance.

Watching the changing thoughts, actions, and words that you use is a blessing. Knowing you are the one with the creative power is priceless.

Your Physical Feelings

Your physical feelings will guide you. Follow all that presents with love. This is the basic level of empathic healing. There are so many levels to this healing technique. This book teaches techniques so that you can be confident as you heal. People healing each other will heal the world. This is a time of great spiritual growth and understanding, and we are only witnessing the beginning of the changes that are going to happen. Please play with this technique. Make it your own and change it, for it will change you. Go deeper into the levels of healing and understanding of concepts of healing with the bodies. The simpler the technique, the easier people will accept the healing. The easier your technique, the easier they will learn and the faster you will advance in your strength and ability.

Trust

Trust is one of the emotions that will help you become a greater healer. The more that you trust in your healing ability, the easier it will be to heal. Building trust is a very easy thing if you understand how to do it. Trust in the way you speak and heal. Look and watch for the changes in those around you. You will learn to accept honor for the changes in people's lives and for their actions. You will be grateful for perceptions and words. Life will become a constant joy and paradise for the future to come. I have been showing others how to see things that they would otherwise miss. I am going to give you these healing steps. I will put forth what should happen with the person you are working on.

These are subtle changes, so you have to look for them.

• **Clean**

As you clean, you will see the person's body language adjust. You will see the shoulders or facial muscles relax. Your body should also relax. Feel for it. Expect it. Create the circumstances for healing in you and those around you by choosing to heal and choosing to have those around you heal consciously or unconsciously. Remember that self-healing should be first and foremost.

• **Protect**

As you protect, you should see other people move farther or closer depending on their unconscious minds. Their body language will change. Their facial expression will also change. This will vary depending on what technique you use.

Protection is a word I use to teach. It is a way for those who have imbalances to assist them in their journey. As you become a greater healer, you will understand that protections will be healed. That which causes a reaction when healed will become blessed. This is the way of the healer.

• **Free**

Freeing the keystones from the bodies is the easiest validation. This is the technique that will give you the most self-trust. The body will relax. Look for the changes. If the keystone has been there a long time, removing it will be like saying goodbye to an old friend, so crying is possible. A person who is standing could become emotional, light-headed, or off-balance. The body will rock back and forth and lean more the harder the person is holding on to a keystone. In time, you will have the pleasure of seeing some take a step forward because you pull so hard at a keystone. The person you are healing may have an emotional reaction without knowing why. This is an excellent indication that you have freed the keystone. It is important to remember to have the keystone turned to energy and dissipate it.

• *Fulfill*

When you are fulfilling, you will see deep contentment on the other's face—a fulfilled look or expression. This step will assist in subsiding people's emotions. You will see that different techniques will present different reactions. I use the technique of using clients' souls to fulfill them. This always gives me the greatest validation by the energy changes and physical relaxation. I do recommend that you try all the techniques and see which one works best for you. Have fun in being guided in this aspect.

Look for validation. It will build your trust in your healing ability and generate more faith in the healing techniques. The greater your trust, the easier seeing and healing will be. Trusting others is one of the reasons we are here. I enjoy watching the movements of my unsuspecting friends as I heal them. It can get comical as you heal. Others will notice what you are doing. To me this is such a source of honor.

Cleansing

There are many great ways to cleanse and heal the physical and etheric bodies. Allow the unlearned lessons to be freed and cleansed. Use the energy of the client and allow it to flow and heal. Look for changing facial expressions as you work this technique. I advocate meditating for personal cleansing. I emphasize the need for elemental healing, which uses Mother Earth to assist us in our walk. We need outdoor time to heal and for our bodies to get the nutrients that they physically require. We need to accept love from our Earth and also to return it to her.

T'ai chi, chi kung, and yoga make use of breathing techniques to help clear issues and imbalances that arise in life. The resulting increased prana and chi flow will free elements that our bodies and aura no longer need. These practices help center and focus the mind, which helps make one a stronger healer. Simply walking or exercising with a controlled breath also works if you are not interested in these types of arts.

There are many tone generators and sounds designed to assist healers in clearing the energy fields. Many discs are available that use these sounds to heal. Look for these online or at your local music store. Ask for recommendations. (See above, p. 44, for my CDs and recommendations.)

Stones and crystals are also used for healing the chakras and the fields. There are many practitioners in this modality of healing. It is a great method for cleansing the full range of the body. The use of oils like lavender helps cleanse the body and fields of unwanted energies and emotions. Such aromatherapies are available in all major health spas or massage clinics. These are just some avenues of healing that you might want to look at. I believe it is important for healers to visit and use other healers. If someone ever tells you, "There is no one clean enough to heal me," I recommend that you find another healer.

Salt

I teach the uses of salt because they are very simple to learn and put into practice. The energetic and physical properties of salt make it an excellent beginner's crystal. During my teachings, salt has been used to assist in protections and in cleanings (physical and energetic). I am not referring to typical tabletop salt, but kosher or pure rock salt. Pure rock salt is available in all areas and markets. It doesn't matter if it comes from a mine or the sea. Each healer will have his or her salt preference. It is readily available and is not expensive.

As salt is a crystal, it can be used with light or any element to amplify the elemental healing. The chemical compound of salt is in all things. It is the beginning of the primordial soup, which is the reason it mimics and amplifies other elements. Salt can be used when you are not sure if there is a crystal for a specific healing. It can be programmed with your intent or filled with a blessing to fulfill or balance the physical and energetic bodies. Salt can also be used to expunge the plasmic energies, thus calming the emotions. It can amplify or mimic oils and herbal treatments.

Salt is used as protection for houses and property by creating permanent barriers. Salt lines around property empowered with intent have been used for thousands of years to protect land from energetic intrusions and imbalances. Salts have been used to cleanse the body in bathing, and in the house as antibacterial cleansers. Salt with lemon drops, rubbing alcohol, and water is an excellent disinfectant for the air, countertops, and doorknobs. Salt has been used in the preparation of blessings for rituals, and has been included in ointments of royalty and priests for many centuries. It is used as medicine in the body and on top of the body. It is a programmable crystal that is used as most crystals are—to intensify and amplify thoughts of intent. Many people use herbs, oils, crystals, spells, and blessings. Yet the use of these items requires extensive knowledge in these disciplines. It takes a lot of time and education to acquire such knowledge. When beginning as a healer, it is nice to have a remedy that is not linked to such extensive knowledge, especially in this busy day and time with so few teachers. Simplicity is the beautiful gift of salt.

Protections

When dealing with energetic entities, or spiritual and emotional battles or issues, the worst thing you will ever encounter is you. I have found that shielding and protections are great but, as you grow and become more knowledgeable, you will no longer need them. The average person might not choose to go so far down the road, which is why I am writing about these simple protections. The first rule is to heal and maintain yourself before healing others. The best protection is the art of self-healing and healing—the art of self-faith.

Protection of the Mind, Body, and Creations

First, keep your personal energy and aura powered up. Exercise regularly to release imbalances and build confidence that supports your willpower. Be mindful of the people you are around for long periods of time. Use and accept love from all things. Let this energy fill all that you are. Pull chi or prana from the earth and the divine to maintain and balance your energy. Use cleaning techniques regularly. Switch the cleaning techniques that you use in order to fully benefit from the practices.

Second, the life you live should be balanced. Try to keep goals and play dates in your mind. While walking with love, fill your future with things that you love to do. Play while you enjoy what you are and have been. In creating future plans, seek out new experiences. Novelty keeps our minds healthy. Keep yourself in good company. Let go of those who need too much of your time. When they are ready, you will be there for them. Remember, you are walking **your** path. All things will cross it: Enjoy them, bless them, and keep following the path.

Third, your consciousness needs to grow and be blessed. Let go of control and the need to know all. When you free things up, you are able to direct with less effort. The thoughts that you think should also be freed. The thoughts that we hear are heard in the conscious and the unconscious minds. These thoughts can control our creation, our lives, and our future. Let them go. Change or correct each thought. Lots of people use positive affirmations to help correct certain thought patterns. Some let the words or pictures of these thoughts turn to smoke and leave the mind and body. Others forgive and honor those thoughts before freeing them. I have taken some to heaven that were too hard to simply let go.

How do you take them to heaven?

I have had energies and thought patterns that were so strong that I could not handle them by myself. I was told by the spirits of ways to heal and honor these energies and patterns I created during my life. I envision each one as a baby: I hold them, I love them as if they were my children, I envision myself walking through the gates of heaven with each child. I see this child transform into a being of this heavenly realm. I return to my body and allow my soul and spirit to fulfill the area the energy has left.

Fourth, be healthy in mind, body, and spirit. Treat yourself as you would a temple or a Stradivarius violin. Be honored. In addition to physically processing what you eat, maintain your spiritual health.

I recommend being gentle when making dietary changes. Start by removing unhealthy foods as you get the feeling or divine direction. Try to eat organic foods and be aware that the meat we eat adds imbalanced emotions into our bodies. All emotions are processed or stored in amino acids. We do not need to acquire bovine fears from their amino acids: Ours are bad enough.

What we drink affects us as much as what we eat. Alcohol depletes our chi, muddles the mind, and puts holes in our auras. Certain types of alcohol are worse than others. Alcohol does have great medicinal properties, but none of them involve its overconsumption. I was taught that medicinal uses involve 2 tablespoons or less—not copious amounts. Alcohol can alter our creative power. It makes us susceptible to others' creations or thoughts changing our esoteric fields.

The water that we drink must also be of high quality. Water makes up almost 80 percent of our bodies.

I understand that finances might be tight when beginning the walk. Food and water can be purified through blessing. The power to bless is in our prayers and words. It is at our fingertips. Bless all that we eat, drink, and are. Bless all that we have been and will be, and all that we meet and will meet. As a parent, I bless my children, others' children, and their infinite offspring.

Fifth, use angels, guides, and totems to protect in all issues of spirit. They understand these things more than our humanity allows us to. Remember that angels do not always look human. Children might see them as monsters. The prophet Ezekiel described cherubim as looking like the Minotaur, having male bodies with oxen heads. Just because you cannot see them doesn't mean that they are not there! Most guides like direction, so have them heal, and bless those who come with ill will and allow them to ascend. Though my totem has fought with me, most guides will not. Angels definitely will not fight with you, as they are protectors. Angels and guides bring the light to give you time and knowledge to heal and prepare.

In these things I advise: *Heal, and then heal and bless all!*

Sixth, use body language as a protector. The way one stands and sits can help protect one's self. It is not my purpose to correct your posture, but slouching and looking down opens the back for accepting others' stuff. To protect the chest and head, cross your arms right over left. This is a subtle defense. It allows you to still accept love and heal others. To cross arms left over right amps up the aura and protects the head and chest, but you are not able to heal or accept others' positive energies. Crossing the legs protects from the abs down to the feet. Cross with knees touching if possible. Again, with right over left you can heal others and pull chi to lower parts of the body. Left over right is defensive and provides stronger protection. Stay away from mirrors when using defensive body-language protections. Mirrors are part of a reflective dimension that allows emotions and energies to become trapped. Have you ever seen a reflection in a pool of water?

This reflection is what a mirror looks like clairvoyantly—then amplified by thousands. I recommend not healing in a room full of mirrors.

Seventh, the clothes you wear can be protective. Silk clothes have great natural properties to protect you from energies and emotions. Bamboo and some organic cottons also have these properties. Bright colors, or "jewel tones," also have protecting abilities from some energies, emotions, and thoughts. Blessing all things that you do and wear is always helpful.

Eighth, using crystals and stones can help protect the bodies. There are so many different techniques in this method that I could write a separate book. Let's begin with jade: a great natural protector. It can be used in chakra charms, bracelets, and necklaces. A chakra charm is seven stones arranged in a particular order. Please do not wear them over the heart chakra, as that will cause an imbalance. Green stones help clean, orange stones help to let go, and gold stones help to balance. Clear stones can intensify effects or channel more power, and pink stones help in accepting and sending love. This is just a short list. Use the stones or crystals depending on the circumstances. Remember—we are healers.

Ninth, amulets can be protective. There are many types of this old-style protection. I recommend that, if you feel you need an amulet, you choose an angelic one and have it blessed by a member of the clergy of your faith. Using amulets blessed by others carries with them their strengths and weakness. You may like the Saints' amulets, or you might want one that heals you and all who come to you. The divine and karmic blessing we all truly need is to be healed at all times and in all dimensions is the greatest blessing. An amulet should be created by you with only love and joy, and then blessed by you and your God or Creator.

Tenth, energetic fires should be used to handle elementals and heavy energy in a room. You may also use golden fire when healing to dissipate the keystones. I have found golden fire to be great when speaking with those whose emotions are running their thought processes.

Shielding

Creating shields is fun and is a part of some healing modalities like vibrational healing. I find it is simplest to teach that shields are flat. They are, but they have an auric feeling to them, so they appear fuzzy when viewed clairvoyantly. Shields are created by intent and formed from energy, plasma, and gaseous material. They are normally created by your dominant hand and placed between you and something or someone.

The shields are programmable, so know what you want yours to do before you create it. That way it won't be patched together. Patched-together shields suffer from imbalances and seem not to last very long. A shield used for healing will stay connected to the hand.

Shields need constant energy. They like to return to you, so make sure they are cleaned when you close them. If you are putting one between you and something or someone, cut the connection between you and the shield when finished so that it does not return.

Please do not walk into a shield that is disconnected, as it will reenter you. When we create shields, we place them between us and others (or fields of energy) that we do not want to accept. If the thing that we shield against is moved or leaves the area, then unconsciously we can be reattracted to our own energy—the shield. If the shield has negative energy attached to it, then the energy will be integrated into you. Dissipate shields into the earth and water when no longer in use. Remember—shields need energy so, once disconnected, they will dissipate in time. Create shields with enough energy to last for however long they need to exist. Please do not add more energy to a shield to make it last longer. Create a new one instead.

When creating a shield, I use colors, but brilliant white or a rainbow is also excellent. I use an intention for what it is to do and for how long it will last. I create anchors and let the energy flow from my hand to fulfill my creation. My shields clean and heal. They are porous and are dissipated by water, so remember that rain can destroy shields. I trust that you will practice creating, using, and testing them before you need one.

Psychic Globes

Psychic globes are also called *psy-balls*. These are created just like shields. Using both hands, create shields and connect them. Most psychic globes are filled with some emotion or healing blessing. I find it easiest to rub my hands together and separate them to the size of globe that I need. Like the shields, these will return if not severed from you. The globe will dissipate in water, or if not connected to another power source. You can place people, things, and thoughts in psychic globes. Be aware that baths and showers can destroy globes that are being used to protect people. Globes are a temporary fix, not a long-term protection. Again, try this mode of protection out in practice before actually relying on it.

The Aura

The aura is the best original shield. We were each born with our aura. It is designed like a wolf's hair: The lovely outer layer shows beauty as well as helping to protect the other aspects of the wolf. The outer hair gets burrs, mud, and blood stuck to it, and is a first defense for the body from personal attack. The inner layer protects from the elements. It is an insulator or thermal barrier. It protects the body from rain and water, as well as protecting and speeding up healing and blood clotting when a wolf has been attacked.

Our aura works the same way energetically. Health rays block unwanted energies. The energies get stuck until we learn to handle or free what is stuck in our health rays. The aura should be strengthened. You can strengthen yours through meditation, through vibrational healing, and by using the cleansing techniques already mentioned.

The better you take care of your body, the stronger your aura is.

There are breathing techniques that strengthen it for a short time while you do them. A belief system can protect a person from all sorts of energies and heal damage without that person ever noticing. This is a trait of religion that is deeply felt and manifest in both the conscious and unconscious.

Light Shielding

Light shielding is a simple technique of using lighted crystals. The crystals' light is shone on pictures or objects that you want to protect. The energy of the light coupled with your intent can prevent an over-influx of unwanted energies on or around the object. When protecting people, their own learned lessons can still attract or react to other energies—meaning that those who are protected by a light shield and get frustrated by their own actions can bring unwanted energies to them, though the imbalance won't last long because of the light shield. Light shields are great for keeping things mellow and smooth while going through life. Green crystals and rose quartz work well for light shields. Try them for yourself and see which color balances you in your path. Each of us is a little different.

Home and Office

Protection for the home and office is the same as for the body and aura. Treat your home and workplace with honor. Do your best to keep them clean and uncluttered. Free yourself and the areas around you from unwanted and broken items. If something has been broken for more than six months, it is going to stay that way. Allow old energy and items to be cleansed from your body, your house, and your life. Keep good energy and air flow through the areas in which you live and work. Try to keep the light bright and use brilliant colors throughout these areas. I recommend evaluating the feng shui in commonly used areas. Place mirrors facing each other at major entrances if you have spirit problems. Use chimes inside and out to help balance the energy in and around the area. When doors open, a bell or chime should go off. This will clear and balance energies that are coming and going.

In these things I advise: *Heal, and then heal and bless all!*

Lavender or purification sprays, and now smudge sprays, can be used in the house and workplace to help keep imbalances to a minimum.

You can burn incense, smudge sticks, Epsom salts, or even frankincense to remove negativity. I have all-healing light shields on my house. There are crystals at the corners of my property that bless all who enter.

I have learned that most protections are aspects of aggression, so I heal and bless all. I teach protections because not all people have the faith in themselves to heal and condone. When negativity is present, I will heal it. If it does not want to be healed, it will leave. *All are welcome when they walk with light and are ready to be healed.*

Understanding

We need to understand what we are doing in order to do it correctly. So, let's look at some basic protocols and see how they flow with our own thoughts. There might be a time you feel like adjusting a protocol. That is fine, as long as you are adding more protection and healing. I prefer that your protection be truly self-healing.

The Techniques of Empathic Healing

- *Balance the aura and chakras*

To protect the physical body, fill the chakras with golden prana. Each chakra naturally contains aspects of gold. The crown chakra has gold that is plasma. It is thick and coats the aura and health rays, allowing more time for healing.

- *Energy balls, shielding*

I have found that a two-layered ball of pink and gold will block or catch imbalances that are present in your fields. It will help evaporate and heal the energy. It also soothes the person letting go of those energies.

- *Emotional display*

If there is an emotional display, cover the person's plasma body with the gold plasma from his or her crown chakra. This will cleanse and start balancing the energies the person accepts and will free, and will assist in calming the emotional body.

- ### *Remember breathing*

Keep the 10-count breathing going. This allows you to separate from emotions and keeps you in the moment.

- ### *Prayer*

I believe in the power of prayer, offered in thought and especially through word, so please try it.

- ### *Protection*

There are times when there is too much energy. Try some of the protective techniques like body language, psychic balls, or tissue salts.

- ### *Remove the keystones*

Use the heart chakra to pull out keystones and see them turn into energy. Allow them to be healed or direct them into a golden fire to completely disintegrate.

- ### *Fulfillment*

Ask that the person's soul and spirit fill the space where the im-balance was removed with his or her essence. Ask that the person always keep it balanced, clean, and divine.

- ### *Golden flame*

Use a golden flame to assist in cleaning the area.

- *Pink light*

Pink light from the heart chakra calms the emotions in the room. In extreme cases, use the crown chakra's golden plasma to fill the plasma body.

- *Validation*

Always watch for the reaction to your healing of those you are working on. You can derive feedback without them knowing.

Let's Get Started Healing

Have you ever entered a building and found a rush of energy or pressure upon entering?

Do you know what to do now?

Here are some hints:

- pray
- protect
- clean
- remove
- fulfill
- validate
- finish the prayer

Here are some protocols I am including based on questions from some of my friends. I hope these will help you adjust the healing that you are already doing. I know they can assist you in your life's journey. I am thankful and honored for you to allow me such an opportunity to assist.

- **Have you ever entered a building and found a rush of energy or pressure upon entering?**

1. Pray as you start to heal. The prayer ends after the healing of the energy or people.

2. Protect yourself. Fill all your chakras with golden energy. You may create a shield or put all that you are in a brilliant white psy-ball.

3. Clean. Fill the room with pink and gold light. In your mind, create a golden fire and allow all the room's energy to flow through the fire to be cleansed.

4. If the building is empty, then step back and feel the new energy to validate it. If the building is occupied with people, then remove the keystones from those present. Remove the keystones in your mind's eye and see them turn to light and disappear. Allow your mind's eye to completely heal and cause the keystones to ascend.

5. Fullfill the empty space where the keystones were present by prayer, brilliant bright light, or golden plasma.

6. Validate. Look for validation by seeing people changing body postures and how they unconsciously react to the energy change. Try to be in the moment when healing by placing the tongue at the roof of your mouth and controlling your breathing.

7. Finish the prayer. Amen.

- **Did the energy leave you as you left the building, or did it shape your whole day?**

1. Prayer or affirmation.

2. Protection should be removed so that you may clean yourself.

3. Clean the bodies of all unbalanced energies. Try to imagine your chakras blowing with gold energy. Have your aura glow with gold energy. If it is difficult then use the liquid gold plasma from the crown chakra above your head.

4. Keystones that attracted this energy should be removed from you.

5. Fulfill the vacant area by asking your soul and spirit to fill the area where the keystones resided.

6. Wait to feel the energy change as validation.

7. Finish the prayer. Amen.

- **Did you notice that it affected others who were not there with you?**

1. Pray that all that you do is divinely done or corrected—that you are balanced, and they are balanced, and all is done for the greater good. Do the healing techniques as part of the prayer.

2. Protect your body by creating a psy-ball of brilliant white light.

3. Clean the aura and chakras of whoever was affected. I would do this by using the liquid gold plasma from the crown chakra thus filling the others' chakras and aura.

4. Keystones should be removed and turned into a dissipating brilliant white light.

5. Fullfill their bodies with one or two of the techniques to fill the empty spaces.

6. Notice the changes as validation.

7. Finish the prayer. Amen.

- **When sitting down to dinner in a restaurant, did you experience the painful feeling of a full stomach? Did the guilt of overeating happen even before you started eating? Did it subside and allow you to enjoy the meal, or did it worsen as you ended the meal?**

1. Pray that the healing is divine and balanced. Remember that protecting, cleaning, and healing are part of the prayer.

2. Protect. In a larger restaurant, you might need to place yourself in a psychic globe.

3. Clean the auras and chakras. To cleanse the room, create a golden fire to cleanse the area.

4. Remove the keystones and see them turn to a brilliant dissipating light.

5. Fulfill the vacant areas inside yourself using your spirit and your soul.

6. For validation, look for people to relax shortly after you complete the protocol.

7. Finish the prayer. Amen.

- **Healing establishments, like hospitals, doctors' offices, and clinics, are places with a lot of sickness and anxiety.**

Has there been a time when you left feeling worse than you did when you arrived? Did that feeling manifest as a physical signal like an itch or a rash?

1. Use prayer or intention that all will be done properly.

2. Protect the aura and chakras. Place yourself inside a psy-ball. You may also choose to use protective body language.

3. Clean by creating a golden fire to cleanse the area.

4. Remove the keystones and turn them into a brilliant dissipating light.

5. Fulfill the vacant areas inside yourself and others.

6. Validate within yourself and others by the energy changes and softening of body features.

7. Finish the prayer. Amen.

Note: Take a salt bath as soon as possible, blessing the salt to cleanse the energy and intent.

- **Have you gone to a funeral service for someone in your interpersonal circle and felt others' grief? Was the grief so real that it clouded your mind?**

Note: It will be helpful to complete a protocol on the building (such as a church or synagogue) prior to arrival. Begin with the prayer. Create a brilliant white psy-ball before you get there. Place the building in golden fire before you arrive to cleanse. Fill the area with a pink light from your heart chakra. Balance your aura and chakras. Remove the keystones; see them change and dissipate and fulfill the vacant areas inside yourself. Validate by feeling the emotions change. Finish the prayer. Amen.

Upon arrival:

1. Pray as you start to heal. The prayer ends after the healing of the energy or people.

2. Protect yourself. Fill all your chakras with golden energy. You may create a shield or put all that you are in a brilliant white psy-ball.

3. Clean. Fill the room with a pink and gold light. In your mind, create a golden fire and allow all the room's energy to flow through the fire to be cleansed.

4. If the building is empty, then step back and feel the new energy to validate it. If the building is occupied with people, then remove the keystones from those present. Remove the keystones in your mind's eye and see them turn to light and disappear. Allow your mind's eye to completely heal and cause the keystones to ascend.

5. Fullfill the empty space where the keystones were present with prayer, brilliant bright light, or golden plasma.

6. Validate. Look for validation by seeing people changing body postures and how they unconsciously react to the energy change. Try to be in the moment when healing by placing your tongue at the roof of your mouth and controlling your breathing.

7. Finish the prayer. Amen.

- ***Has there been a violent injury or attack that someone else endured but you have a physical reaction to, such as grief or anger?***

1. Pray that all healing be done divinely and all emotions be balanced quickly.

2. Protect. Put yourself and the person you are healing in two separate brilliant white psy-balls.

3. Clean. Create a large golden fire with green tips to cleanse the energy and the emotions. Pull the energy into the fire and radiate a pink glow from your heart chakra that surrounds all. Cleanse the aura and chakras for all people affected.

4. Remove the keystones in all affected and see them turn into a brilliant dissipating light.

5. Fulfill the vacant areas using one of the appropriate techniques.

6. Validate by the people's calming reactions and look for their bodies to sway.

7. Finish the prayer. Amen.

- ***Have you ever wanted to pay for someone's life choices and thoughts? For instance, at a store you notice that the person ahead of you does not have enough money. Would you pay for that person in order to alleviate the pain of embarrassment and to relieve pressure in your own body?***

1. Pray that all energies are healed divinely.

2. Protect yourself by strengthening your aura (fill the chakras with plasmic gold from your crown chakra and pulse it throughout your aura).

3. Clean. Use a 10-count breathing technique to clean yourself.

4. Remove the keystone that created the embarrassment in your emotions. Remove the keystone in the other person that has created a block to financial abundance. See the keystones turn into a brilliant dissipating light.

5. Fulfill both your body and the other person's with a brilliant white light or ask your spirit and soul to fulfill you and the other's spirit and soul to fulfill him or her.

6. Validate by your own emotions calming.

7. Finish the prayer. Amen.

- **Do you see people struggle with learning, watching them step out of the box from their life circumstances at work or school?**

1. Pray that all energies are healed divinely.

2. Protect yourself by strengthening your aura (fill the chakras with plasmic gold from your crown chakra and pulse it throughout your aura).

3. Clean. Create a golden fire and clean the emotions and energy of the room.

4. Remove the keystone that created the embarrassment in yourself. Remove the keystone in the other person that has

created a block to wisdom and knowledge. See the keystones turn into a brilliant dissipating light.

5. Fulfill both your body and the other person's with a brilliant white light or ask your spirit and soul to fulfill you and the other's spirit and soul to fulfill him or her.

6. Validate by your own emotions calming.

7. Finish the prayer. Amen.

- **Have you felt someone else's physical pain, such as a headache or backache, when you are nearby?**

1. Pray that all energies are healed divinely.

2. Protect yourself by strengthening your aura (fill the chakras with plasma gold from your crown chakra and pulse it throughout your aura).

3. Clean. Create a golden fire and clean the emotions and energy of the painful area.

4. Remove the keystone in the other person and see the keystone turn into a brilliant dissipating light.

5. Fulfill—by asking the person's spirit or soul to fulfill him or her.

6. Validate by the other's reduction of pain.

7. Finish the prayer. Amen.

- **Have you felt the pain of a pet, or a wounded wild animal's panic or other emotions?**

1. Pray that all energies are healed divinely.

2. Protect yourself by strengthening your aura (fill the chakras with plasmic gold from your crown chakra and pulse it throughout your aura).

3. Clean. Create a golden fire and clean the emotions and energy of the painful area.

4. Remove the keystone in the pet and see the keystone turn into a brilliant dissipating light.

5. Fulfill—by asking the pet's spirit or soul to fulfill him or her.

6. Validate by the animal's reduction of pain.

7. Finish the prayer. Amen.

- ***Does the sound of a baby crying impart to you the mother's panic or the baby's unease and confusion?***

1. Pray that all energies are healed divinely.

2. Protect yourself by strengthening your aura (fill the chakras with gold plasma from your crown chakra and pulse it throughout your aura).

3. Clean. Create a golden fire and clean the emotions and energy of child and yourself. Radiate into the room a pink glow from your heart chakra that permeates all.

4. Remove the keystones in the child, yourself, and those affected. See the keystone turn into a brilliant dissipating light.

5. Fulfill—by asking the person's spirit or soul to fulfill him or her. Ask your soul or spirit to fulfill you.

6. Validate by the calming of the energy.

7. Finish the prayer. Amen.

- **What about happy events like an amusement-park visit or a wedding? Do you feel the excitement of the rides or fear boiling?**

1. Pray that all energies are healed divinely.

2. Protect yourself by strengthening your aura (fill the chakras with plasmic gold from your crown chakra and pulse it throughout your aura).

3. Clean. Create a golden fire and clean the emotions and energy of the people.

4. Remove the keystone in yourself and others. See the keystones turn into a brilliant dissipating light.

5. Fulfill both your body and the other person's with a brilliant white light or ask your spirit and soul to fulfill you and the other's spirit and soul to fulfill him or her.

6. Validate by your own emotions calming.

7. Finish the prayer. Extinguish the fire. Amen.

- **Are you around friends and family knowing they are drinking or using drugs excessively, including over-the-counter and prescription drugs?**

1. Pray that all energies are healed divinely.

2. Protect. Put yourself in a psy-ball.

3. Clean. Create a golden fire and clean the emotions and energy of the room.

4. Remove the keystone in yourself that is affected. Remove any keystones present within the person that have created the

imbalance. See the keystones turn into a brilliant dissipating light.

5. Fulfill both your body and the other person's with a brilliant white light or ask your spirit and soul to fulfill you and the other's spirit and soul to fulfill him or her.

6. Validate by feeling the energy change inside of you.

7. Finish the prayer. Extinguish the fire. Amen.

- **At work, do you feel the energy when coworkers get upset about something?**

1. Pray that all energies are healed divinely.

2. Protect. Put yourself in a psy-ball.

3. Clean. Create a golden fire and clean the emotions and energy of the room. Exhale a pink glow that fills the room from your heart chakra.

4. Remove the keystone in yourself that is affected. Remove any keystones present within your coworkers that have created the imbalance. See the keystones turn into a brilliant dissipating light.

5. Fulfill both your body and the other person's with a brilliant white light or ask your spirit and soul to fulfill you and the other's spirit and soul to fulfill him or her.

6. Validate by feeling the energy change inside of you.

7. Finish the prayer. Extinguish the fire. Amen.

- **Do you need to talk or deal with people in authority?**

1. Pray that all energies are healed divinely.

2. Protect. Put yourself in a psy-ball.

3. Clean. Create a golden fire and clean the emotions and energy of the area. Exhale a pink glow that fills the room from your heart chakra.

4. Remove the keystone in yourself that is affected. See the keystones turn into a brilliant dissipating light.

5. Fulfill both your body and the other person's with a brilliant white light or ask your spirit and soul to fulfill you and the other's spirit and soul to fulfill him or her.

6. Validate by feeling the energy change inside of you.

7. Finish the prayer. Extinguish the fire. Amen.

- **What about when people complain or use negative words?**

1. Pray that all energies are healed divinely.

2. Protect. Use protective body language.

3. Clean. Create a golden fire and clean the emotions and energy of the room. Send a pink light from your heart chakra to those being negative.

4. Remove the keystone in yourself that is affected. Remove any keystones present within the complaining or negative people that have created the imbalance. See the keystones turn into a brilliant dissipating light.

5. Fulfill both your body and the others' with a brilliant white

light or ask your spirit and soul to fulfill you and the others' spirit and soul to fulfill them.

6. Validate by feeling the energy change inside of you.

7. Finish the prayer. Extinguish the fire. Amen.

Note: You should do your best to change the subject to something positive or walk away. Watch your thoughts. Do not agree with the negative words; reword them in your head.

- **What if someone you have a relationship with is upset and vents to you, causing you to feel worse than before your partner vented?**

1. Pray that all energies are healed divinely.

2. Protect. Use protective body language.

3. Clean. Create a golden fire and clean the emotions and energy of the room. Send a pink light, which you may alternate with gold light from the heart chakra.

4. Remove the keystone in yourself that is affected. Remove any keystones present within your partner that have created the imbalance. See the keystones turn into a brilliant dissipating light.

5. Fulfill both your body and your partner's with a brilliant white light or ask your spirit and soul to fulfill you and the other's spirit and soul to fulfill him or her.

6. Validate by feeling the energy change inside of you.

7. Finish the prayer. Extinguish the fire. Amen.

Note: Examine your thoughts. Understand that the things being said are the issues that your partner needs to have healed—even if the words being said are about you. Stay in the moment. Use the breathing technique. You may want to balance your aura, body, and minds multiple times.

- **Do you allow yourself to spend too much time reflecting on past relationships, and allowing your mind to start running in unhealthy patterns?**

1. Pray that all energies are healed divinely.

2. Protect. Fill your chakras and aura with a brilliant white light.

3. Clean. Create a golden fire with green tips to clean your emotions.

4. Remove the keystones in yourself that are affecting you. See the keystones turn into a brilliant dissipating light.

5. Fulfill your body with a brilliant white light or ask your spirit or soul to fulfill you.

6. Validate by feeling the energy change inside of you.

7. Finish the prayer. Extinguish the fire. Amen.

Note: Watch your thoughts. Quickly fill the words, thoughts, or pictures with white light, and say "heal" three times. Keep doing this until the mind changes the subject. Try taking on a project that takes a lot of mental effort, or do some exercise to release endorphins.

- **Do others sometimes take what you say in a way you did not mean? Are the resulting topics sometimes uncomfortable?**

1. Pray that all energies are healed divinely.

2. Protect. Fill your chakras and aura with a brilliant white light.

3. Clean. Create a golden fire and clean the emotions and energy of the room. Send a pink light from the heart chakra.

4. Remove the keystone in yourself that is affected. Remove any keystones present within the people that have created the imbalance. See the keystones turn into a brilliant dissipating light.

5. Fulfill both your body and the others' with a brilliant white light or ask your spirit and soul to fulfill you and the others' spirit and soul to fulfill them.

6. Validate by feeling the energy change inside of you.

7. Finish the prayer. Extinguish the fire. Amen.

- **Do you find yourself helping someone with something that person does not want to heal?**

1. Pray that all energies are healed divinely.

2. Protect. Fill your chakras and aura with a brilliant white light.

3. Clean. Fill the other's chakras with a gold and white light. Fill his or her mind with a brilliant white light.

4. Remove the keystone in yourself that is affected. Remove any keystones present within the person that have created the imbalance. See the keystones turn into a brilliant dissipating light.

5. Fulfill both your body and the other person's with a brilliant white light or ask your spirit and soul to fulfill you and the other's spirit and soul to fulfill him or her.

6. Validate by feeling the energies calm or the other person accepting the healing.

7. Finish the prayer. Extinguish the fire. Amen.

Note: Heal and you will not have to speak about it.

- **Are you working with someone defensive?**

1. Pray that all energies are healed divinely.

2. Protect. Fill your chakras and aura with a brilliant white light.

3. Clean. Fill the defensive person's chakras with a gold and white light. Send a pink light from the heart chakra to the person who is defensive. See his or her aura turn pink in your mind's eye.

4. Remove the keystone in yourself that is affected. Remove any keystones present within the defensive person that have created the imbalance. See the keystones turn into a brilliant dissipating light.

5. Fulfill both your body and the defensive person's with a brilliant white light or ask your spirit and soul to fulfill you and the other's spirit and soul to fulfill him or her.

6. Validate by feeling the energies calm.

7. Finish the prayer. Extinguish the fire. Amen.

- **What if you have a hard time keeping your gold flames around you when someone in your interpersonal circle is irritated?**

1. Pray that all energies are healed divinely.

2. Protect. Use protective body language. Put yourself in a brilliant white psy-ball.

3. Clean by putting those around you in a psy-ball of pink and gold.

4. Remove the keystones in yourself that are affecting you. Remove any keystones present within the person that have created the imbalance. See the keystones turn into a brilliant dissipating light.

5. Fulfill both your body and the irritated person's with a brilliant white light or ask your spirit and soul to fulfill you and the irritated one's spirit and soul to fulfill him or her.

6. Validate by feeling the energies calm and a strengthening aura.

7. Finish the prayer. Extinguish the fire. Amen.

Note: If your imagination or intention is not working, use *your word.* Try to think it in your mind then say out loud. Here is an example. Think "green fire," then say it out loud. Think and say "cleanse minds and auras" out loud. Verbally state that the keystones in both you and others are removed. Say, "integrate the keystones perfectly," and you will be fulfilled by your own soul—as are we all. One's word spoken out loud is more powerful than most people could imagine.

Remember to follow steps 1–7:

Pray, protect, clean, remove keystones, fulfill, validate, and finish the prayer.

- **Have you gone out to lunch with a friend who had a problem? You sat and listened and, when lunch was** *over, your friend felt so much better as you walked away with pain in your heart? Without realizing it, you took your friend's emotional pain and issues.*

After reading this book, my question to you is: How would you heal the situation?

Congratulations! You are a balanced and knowledge-able empathic healer!

Glossary

affirmation. A way to change your thought patterns and the energy vibrations in your bodies. A prayer to your higher self or your divine self (the I AM).

amulet. An item that is intentionally charged to create a certain barrier or energetic output.

aura(s). The energetic output of your bodies coexisting in your physical body.

auric fields. Layers of vibrations and frequencies that pertain to different aspects and insights into your life.

chakra. An energy vortex that pulls in energy and expels energy into all of your bodies.

chi (qi). Energy that flows through our body as easy as breath. It permeates our thoughts, minds, and actions.

clairaudience. The ability to hear energy, vibrations, and frequencies. (*Cf.* **clairvoyance**.)

clairvoyance. The ability to see energy, vibrations, and frequencies. (*Cf.* **clairaudience**.)

crystals. Nature's pre-programmed energetic healers.

energy. Equivalent to **prana** or **chi**. The life-force energy that flows through our body.

empathic. Able to feel other people's emotions, pains, and sometimes thoughts.

esoteric. Rarely seen; understood by few.

fulfill. As used in this book, a concept to fill the area where the keystones formerly resided. There are many techniques to fulfillment.

health rays. Cilia-like lines that are part of your aura. They extend from your energetic body from $1/16$ inch away to many feet out.

intention. The mind's eye to send energy to a certain point with thought, words and actions.

keystone. An issue in your life that blocks or resists healing and prevents us from moving forward. It attracts or repulses things in your life.

meditation. A way to calm your body, quiet your mind, and create joy in your life.

mind. Another word for ego, id, and superego, all rolled into one.

plasma. A type of liquid energy that exists in and out of the body.

prana. Another word for **chi**. An energy that exists in the body.

prayer. A way to get assistance in the road we choose for our life by asking divine spirits to assist.

protection. A word that has an aggressive tone; I use it as an aspect to assist in your healing. As you become a stronger healer, your protection shall become healing.

psy-ball, psychic globe. Ball created by energy to encompass something and programmed for a certain output.

Index

alcohol 25, 55
  rubbing 51
amulets 57–58
aura 15–18, 23, 29, 49, 53,
    56, 60–61, 63, 64,
    66–83 *passim*
  human 27
  prayer and 43
  stress and 7
balance 17–18, 19, 41, 48, 49, 53,
    57, 65, 67, 76, 80
  aura and chakras 63, 69, 79
  bodies 23, 24, 50
  emotions 4, 17, 37, 71
  energy 53, 62
  mind 29
bodies see energetic body
chakra(s) 12, 14–18, 72
  balance 63
  charms 57
  crown 18, 23, 24, 26, 30, 36,
    37, 44, 63, 65, 67, 72, 73,
    74, 75 see also plasma,
    golden
  dan tien 26
  earth 30
  foot 14, 15
  heart 25, 26, 29, 34, 41
    and charms 57

  and keystones 64
  and pink light 38–39,
    65, 69, 71, 74, 76, 77,
    78, 80, 81
  shielding 26
  knee 14, 15
  major 14, 15
  minor 14
  root 26
  solar plexus 25
chi (prana) 12, 13, 14, 15, 17, 23,
    24, 33, 49, 56, 63
  alcohol and 55
  and protections 53
clairaudience 36, 42
clairvoyance 30, 34, 35, 36, 42,
    57, 58
  clairvoyant eye(s) 15, 36
empathic healing 1–3, 7–9, 13,
    24, 46
  basics 6–7
  clairvoyance, relationship
    to 36
  examples 1–2
  heart chakra 34
    shielding 26
  teaching with visual
    markers 35
  techniques 13, 14, 46, 48, 63ff

energetic body (bodies)   9,
     11–13, 17, 18, 25–26
   atomic   13, 24
   etheric   12, 13–14, 15, 16,
     25, 49
   gaseous   12, 13, 24
   liquid   12, 13
   plasmic   13
   salt and   50
   subatomic   12, 24
   superetheric   12, 24
energy balls   see psychic globes
energy fields   see fields, energy
esoteric fields   see fields,
     esoteric
fields   19, 27, 34, 63   see also
     aura
   energy   15, 18, 49, 59
   esoteric   15, 16, 55
   etheric   9
health rays   16–18, 23, 27, 60, 63
keystones   19–23, 26, 30, 34–38,
     43, 44, 45, 47–48, 58, 64,
     66–82 *passim*
maladies   4–5
plasma   12–13, 17
   golden   23, 24, 37, 38, 44, 63,
     65, 67, 70 72, 73, 74, 75
prana   see chi

psy-balls   see psychic globes
psychic globes (psy-balls, energy
     balls)   59–60, 63, 64, 66,
     68, 69, 70, 71, 75, 76, 77,
     81, 82
prayer   21, 30–31, 36, 38, 43, 55,
     64, 65–82 *passim*
protection   3, 7, 15, 17, 18,
     23–25, 27, 38, 47,
     50, 52–62, 63, 64,
     65–82 *passim*
salt   27, 50–51, 69
   Epsom salts   62
   tissue salts   64
shielding   23, 25–27, 34, 38, 39,
     53, 59, 60, 66, 70   see
     also psychic globes
   light shields   61, 62

About the Author

Daniel Staite lives outside of Austin, Texas, with his wife and two children. He served in the Marine Corps and is a lifelong student of the martial arts including kung fu, t'ai chi, and jiu jitsu.

Daniel began his training as healer and prophet under the tutelage of his Indian grandmother 40 years ago. His passion for elemental healing was the inspiration for his CDs and this book. He believes that the manifestation of joy and love should be easier for all people. He invites you to enjoy the experience of healing yourself and those around you.

More DANIEL
from STAITE

Meditation CDs
from Blue Oak Record Group
Meditation for Healing (DS 0901)
Meditation for Interpersonal Relations (DS 0902)

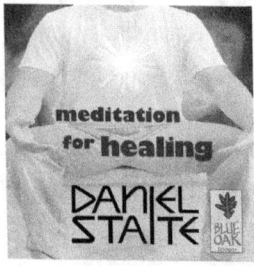 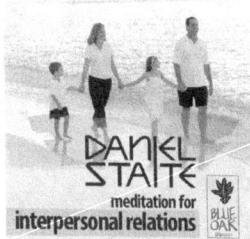

Available online at **www.cdbaby.com/danielstaite** or at the iTunes store. More info and future releases at **www.corneroak.com/blueoak**.

Web site
The Healing State
www.thehealingstate.com
Dedicated to all seeking emotional, spiritual, mental, physical,
or financial healing for themselves

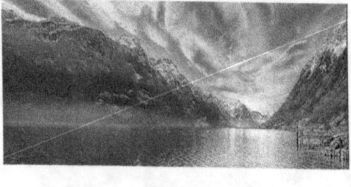

and others. For shamans, masters, and those just trying to be fruitful and fulfilled in their own lives.

Cookbook
Best Gluten Free Friends Cookbook
Ann Davila, Daniel Staite, Jeanie Steuer, Nancy Willard
www.amazon.com, search "daniel staite"
or follow the link at **www.corneroak.com/staite**
Spirited salads, breads you can live with, heartwarming
soups, lovable snacks, simple sides, meals of suste-
nance, grand-finale desserts.

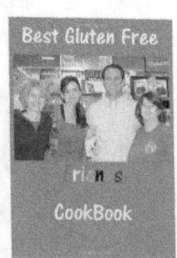

www.ingramcontent.com/pod-product-compliance
Lightning Source LLC
Chambersburg PA
CBHW062040280526
45788CB00003B/1053